Table of Contents

Introduction

Hemochromatosis is a condition in which the body absorbs too much of the iron consumed from food. This over absorption leads to high levels of iron in the blood that the body can't get rid of. When this iron is deposited into vital organs, such as the liver, heart, and pancreas, it can cause oxidative stress and long-term damage. For people with hemochromatosis, there are different ways to reduce the amount of iron in the body. One of the methods of keeping iron levels low is through dietary modifications. Let's look at the best diet for hemochromatosis, including foods to eat, foods to avoid, supplements to take, and recipes to try.

It's about more than just how much iron you consume

In a broad sense, the best diet for hemochromatosis involves foods low in iron. However, there are various circumstances that can affect how much iron is absorbed from the foods you eat. Here are some dietary factors that may affect the way your body absorbs iron:

• Heme vs. nonheme iron. There are two types of dietary iron: heme and nonheme. Heme iron is found in meat and seafood. Nonheme is found in plants, meat, seafood, and fortified products. Heme iron is more bioavailable than nonheme iron, meaning that it's more easily absorbed by your body.

• Vitamin C. Vitamin C, or ascorbic acid, enhances the bioavailability of nonheme iron. In addition, meat and seafood can also enhance the absorption of nonheme iron.

• Calcium. Various forms of calcium may decrease the bioavailability of both heme and nonheme iron.

• Phytate and polyphenols. Phytate, or phytic acid, is a compound found in grains and legumes that decreases the absorption of iron. Other compounds in plant foods, known as polyphenols, can also decrease iron absorption.

As you can see, avoiding iron-rich foods is only one element of the best diet for hemochromatosis. There are other items, such as the other nutrients in the foods you eat, that can affect your iron absorption.

What is hemochromatosis

Hemochromatosis is a condition where there is too much iron in the body. Most commonly, this occurs due to faulty genes (usually the HFE gene) in iron regulation. When the disease is due to genetic reasons, it is called Hereditary Hemochromatosis (HH). HH is a lifelong (chronic) disease, while other causes of hemochromatosis — too many blood transfusions, diseases that destroy red blood cells, and taking too many iron supplements — resolve with treatment and time.

Symptoms include liver disease, diabetes, skin discoloration, arthritis, and heart failure. However, if treated, these symptoms can be mostly or completely avoided. Hemochromatosis can be diagnosed with blood testing. It is treated by medical phlebotomy (bloodletting), chelating agents (metal binders), and a low-iron diet.

Main symptoms

In cases of HH, symptoms typically manifest in midlife. For non-hereditary cases, symptoms can manifest at any time. The hallmark symptoms include:

• High blood sugar (hyperglycemia): Symptoms include thirst, fatigue, nausea/vomiting, and frequent urination.

• Skin bronzing: The increased iron deposits in the skin, leading to a bronze-colored pigmentation.

• Cirrhosis: Replacement of normal liver cells with fibrous bands, causing liver damage and possibly liver failure.

Other symptoms

Other, less common symptoms include:

• Arthritis

• Fatigue

• Erectile dysfunction

Complications

Complications of hemochromatosis include the following, which can affect various body systems.

• Diabetes: The insulin-producing cells of the pancreas are damaged and can lead to high blood sugar that may require injectable insulin if the damage is extensive.

• Hepatocellular carcinoma: Cancer of the liver.

• Cardiomyopathy: This is damage to the heart muscle which can lead to heart failure (inadequate pumping of blood to the body).

• Pericarditis: Inflammation of the sac surrounding the heart leading to chest pain.

• Hypogonadism: Insufficient production of hormones by the ovaries or testicles, leading to decreased levels of estrogen and testosterone, respectively.

• Hypopituitarism: Insufficient production of hormones by the pituitary gland.

Hemochromatosis can be caused by either genetic or environmental causes. Both mechanisms of the disease lead to elevated blood levels of iron. It is the increased amount of iron that causes the symptoms of hemochromatosis because the excess iron gets deposited in almost every tissue in the body.

Genetic causes

Hereditary hemochromatosis (HH) is one of the most common diseases of white people. Most commonly, hemochromatosis is caused by inheriting a genetic mutation (error) that causes the body to mishandle the iron it receives from food. There are many possible mutations that can cause hereditary hemochromatosis, but the majority of people with HH have a mutation called C2823Y in the gene called HFE. This causes a two- to three-fold increased absorption of iron from food. The best way to diagnose the disease is through a liver biopsy. However, MRI images, genetic testing and laboratory testing can also help the diagnosis. There are, however, other genetic causes of HH that do not result from mutation of the HFE gene:

• African iron overload

• Juvenile hemochromatosis

• Neonatal hemochromatosis

• Aceruloplasminemia

• Transfusional siderosis

• Environmental causes

The non-genetic causes of hemochromatosis are:

• Excessive dietary iron intake: This includes taking too many iron supplement pills.

• Excessive blood transfusions

• Chronic dialysis

• Chronic liver disease: This can occur hepatitis C, alcoholism, or fatty liver disease.

• Porphyria cutanea tarda

• Sideroblastic anemia

If treatment begins early, people can expect to lead a normal life with normal life-expectancy. However, if treatment is delayed until after diabetes, cirrhosis, hypogonadism, or hypopituitarism develop, these processes cannot be reversed.

Therapeutic phlebotomy (bloodletting)

One of the mainstay treatments of hemochromatosis is therapeutic phlebotomy (bloodletting), which is when blood is removed from the body. This serves to decrease overall iron stores and is a generally safe and effective practice. Therapeutic phlebotomy is generally performed once the iron level is high enough. Typically, one unit of blood is taken per week initially until the blood iron level is slightly below normal. Thereafter, therapeutic phlebotomy is performed as needed depending on the blood iron level. This method of treatment requires routine blood laboratory testing to ensure that an appropriate amount of blood is being removed from the body. On average, men require therapeutic phlebotomy twice as often as women do. It may take more than a year to normalize body iron levels.

Medication

For people who cannot receive therapeutic phlebotomy, a drug called an iron chelator can be given. Deferoxamine, an iron chelator, acts to bind iron, soaking it up from the blood and allowing it to be removed in the urine and feces.

Dietary changes

People with hemochromatosis should never take iron supplement pills. You should also restrict your intake of vitamin C. In addition, you should limit your consumption of red meat since it has a high iron content. You should also avoid alcohol since it increases the chance of liver damage in people with hemochromatosis. Some advise the avoidance of raw shellfish since it can cause an infection in people with hemochromatosis.

The genetic causes of HH cannot be prevented because they are inherited. However, there are certain measures that can be taken to lessen the severity of the disease. For example, people with HH should never take iron supplements and should follow the dietary modifications listed in the previous section. Regular care from a physician who treats HH should be obtained in order to prevent the permanent complications from HH.

On the other hand, the environmental causes of hemochromatosis are more preventable. For each type of environmental cause, the prevention strategy is given below:

• Excessive dietary iron intake: Avoid excessive iron supplements.

• Excessive blood transfusions: Physicians should monitor and limit the amount of blood you receive or consider giving you iron chelators.

• Chronic liver disease: The underlying cause of liver disease should be managed.

• Porphyria cutanea tarda: This will likely be treated with bloodletting and medication.

• Sideroblastic anemia: This will likely be treated with pyridoxine and iron chelation will be used if needed.

If you receive a diagnosis of HH, then it may be prudent for your relatives to undergo genetic testing to check for the disease before symptoms begin.

Foods to eat when you have hemochromatosis

Fruits and vegetables

With hemochromatosis, excess iron increases oxidative stress and free radical activity, which can damage your DNA.

Antioxidants play an important role in protecting your body from the damage caused by oxidative stress. Fruits and vegetables are a great source of many antioxidants, such as vitamin E, vitamin C, and flavonoids. Many of the recommendations for hemochromatosis will warn you to stay away from vegetables high in iron. This may not always be necessary.

Vegetables that are high in iron, such as spinach and other leafy greens, contain only nonheme iron. Nonheme iron is less easily absorbed than heme iron, making vegetables a good choice. Talk to your doctor or dietitian if you have concerns.

Grains and legumes

Grains and legumes contain substances that inhibit iron absorption — specifically, phytic acid.

For many people, a diet high in grains may place them at risk for mineral deficiencies, such as calcium, iron, or zinc.

However, for people with hemochromatosis, this phytic acid can help to keep the body from overabsorbing iron from foods.

Eggs

Eggs are a source of nonheme iron, so are they fine to eat on a hemochromatosis diet? Actually, the answer is yes — due to a phosphoprotein in the egg yolk called phosvitin.

Research has shown that phosvitin may inhibit the absorption of iron, among other minerals. In one animal study, researchers found that rats fed with a yolk protein had lower iron absorption than rats given soy or casein protein.

Tea and coffee

Both tea and coffee contain polyphenolic substances called tannins, also known as tannic acid. The tannins in tea and coffee inhibit iron absorption. This makes these two popular beverages a great addition to your diet if you have hemochromatosis.

Lean protein

Protein is an important part of a healthy diet. Many dietary sources of protein do contain iron. However, this doesn't mean that you have to cut meat out of your diet completely. Instead, plan your meals around protein sources that are lower in iron, such as turkey, chicken, tuna, and even deli meat.

Foods to avoid when you have hemochromatosis

Excess red meat

Red meat can be a healthy part of a well-rounded diet if eaten in moderation. The same may be said for those with hemochromatosis.

Red meat is a source of heme iron, meaning that the iron is more easily able to be absorbed by the body. If you continue to eat red meat, consider eating only two to three servings per week. You can pair it with foods that decrease the absorption of iron.

Raw seafood

Although seafood itself doesn't contain a dangerous amount of iron, there's something in raw shellfish that might be more concerning.

Vibrio vulnificus is a type of bacteria present in coastal waters and can infect the shellfish in these areas. Older research has suggested that iron plays an integral role in the spread of V. vulnificus.

For people with high levels of iron, such as those with hemochromatosis, it's important to avoid raw shellfish.

Foods rich in vitamins A and C

Vitamin C, or ascorbic acid, is one of the most effective enhancers of iron absorption. Although vitamin C is a necessary part of a healthy diet, you may want to be aware of vitamin C-rich foods and eat them in moderation. In addition, vitamin A has also been shown to increase the absorption of iron in human studies.

Note that many leafy green vegetables contain vitamin C, vitamin A, and iron. However, since nonheme iron present in vegetables isn't as easily absorbed, the benefits seem to outweigh the risks.

Fortified foods

Fortified foods have been fortified with nutrients. Many fortified foods contain high amounts of vitamins and minerals such as calcium, zinc, and iron. If you have hemochromatosis, eating iron-rich fortified foods may increase your blood iron levels. Check the iron content on nutrition labels before you eat these types of foods.

Excess alcohol

Alcohol consumption, especially chronic alcohol consumption, can damage the liver. Iron overload in hemochromatosis can also cause or worsen liver damage, so alcohol should only be consumed moderately. If you have any type of liver condition due to hemochromatosis, you shouldn't consume alcohol at all, as this could further damage your liver.

Supplements

There aren't many recommendations for additional supplements when you have hemochromatosis. This is because research is limited on dietary interventions for this condition. Still, you should avoid or be careful with the following supplements:

• Iron. As you can imagine, taking iron when you have hemochromatosis can place you at risk for extremely high levels of iron in the body.

• Vitamin C. Although vitamin C is a popular supplement for iron-deficiency anemia, it should be avoided in those with hemochromatosis. You can consume your daily recommended value of vitamin C through whole fruits and vegetables instead.

• Multivitamins. If you have hemochromatosis, you should take multivitamin or multimineral supplements with caution. They may contain high amounts of iron, vitamin C, and other nutrients that enhance iron absorption. Always check the label and consult with your doctor.

Recipes

Vegetable Quiche

Ingredients

• 1 tbsp. olive oil

• 1/2 cup green onion, chopped

• 1/2 cup onion, chopped

• 1/2 cup zucchini, chopped

• 1 cup spinach

• 3 eggs, beaten

• 1/2 cup milk

• 1 1/2 cups shredded cheese

• 1 deep dish pie crust, precooked

Directions

• Preheat the oven to 350°F (177°C).

• In a large skillet, heat the olive oil. Add the green onion, onion, and zucchini. Cook for 5 minutes.

• Add the spinach. Cook for an additional 2 minutes. Remove the cooked vegetables from the skillet and set aside.

• In a mixing bowl, whisk the eggs, milk, half of the cheese, and salt and pepper to taste.

• Pour the egg mixture into the pie crust. Top with the remainder of the shredded cheese.

• Bake for 40–45 minutes, or until the eggs are cooked throughout.

Turkey Chili

Ingredients

• 1 tbsp. olive oil

• 1 lb. ground turkey

• 1 large onion, chopped

• 2 cups chicken broth

• 1 (28-ounce) can red tomatoes, crushed

• 1 (16-ounce) can kidney beans, drained and rinsed

• 2 tbsp. chili powder

• 1 tbsp. garlic, chopped

• 1/2 tsp. each cayenne, paprika, dried oregano, cumin, salt, and pepper

Directions

• In a large pot over medium heat, heat olive oil. Add the ground turkey and cook until browned. Add the chopped onion and cook until tender.

• Add the chicken broth, tomatoes, and kidney beans. Add remaining ingredients and stir thoroughly.

• Bring to a boil then reduce heat to low. Cover and simmer for 30 minutes.

Blueberry Salad with Grilled Turmeric Chicken

INGREDIENTS

• 1 pound (450 g) chicken breasts, cut into 1-inch (2.5-cm) thick strips

• Salt and black pepper as needed

• 1 teaspoon ground turmeric

• ½ teaspoon curry powder

• 5 tablespoons (75 ml) olive oil, divided

• 4 cups (120 g) coarsely chopped butterhead lettuce

• 1 cup (144 g) fresh blueberries

• ½ cup (60 g) pecan halves

• 2 ounces (58 g) feta or blue cheese, crumbled

INSTRUCTIONS

• Season the chicken with the salt and pepper.

• In a small bowl, make a paste with the turmeric, curry powder, and 1 tablespoon (15 ml) of the oil. Coat the chicken strips in the paste and set them aside.

• Preheat the grill, electric grill, or stovetop grill pan to medium-high heat (400°F [200°C]). Spray it with cooking spray then add the chicken and cook 5 to 7 minutes per side (or 5 to 7 minutes total with a two-sided electric grill) until the chicken reaches an internal temperature of 165°F (74°C).

• Fill 4 salad bowls with the lettuce and coat it with the remaining 4 tablespoons (60 ml) oil, then top with the chicken strips, blueberries, pecans, and cheese.

Buttermilk Green Tea Roasted Chicken

INGREDIENTS

- 1 teaspoon dried thyme

- 1 teaspoon dried sage

- 1 teaspoon ground mustard seeds

- 1 tablespoon (2 g) dried rosemary

- 2 teaspoons (10 g) salt

- 1 teaspoon ground black pepper

- 2 tablespoons (30 ml) honey

- 1 cup (240 ml) buttermilk

- 1 cup (240 ml) brewed green tea chilled

- 2 pounds (900 g) skin-on, bone-in chicken pieces (breasts, legs, and so on)

INSTRUCTIONS

- In a medium bowl, mix together the thyme, sage, mustard seeds, rosemary, salt, and pepper. Stir in the honey, buttermilk, and green tea. Place the chicken and the marinade in a large resealable bag or lidded bowl then refrigerate for at least 2 hours and up to 24 hours.

• Preheat the oven to 425°F (220°C). Line a medium roasting tray with foil. Let the excess marinade drip off the chicken pieces and place the pieces on the prepared roasting tray. Bake for approximately 30 minutes, until the chicken skin is crispy and the meat reaches an internal temperature of 165°F (74°C).

Split Pea and Mint Soup

INGREDIENTS

• ⅓ cup (66 g) dried green split peas

• 3½ cups (840 ml) water plus 1-2 Tbsp extra water

• 1 tablespoon (15 ml) extra virgin olive oil

• 2 medium onions coarsely chopped

• 3 cloves garlic minced

• 5 cups (1.2 L) vegetable stock

• ½ teaspoon salt plus more as needed

• ¼ teaspoon black pepper plus more as needed

• 2 green tea bags

• 10 ounces (280 g) fresh or frozen green peas

• 10 to 20 fresh mint leaves plus more as needed

• Milk or cream optional, to taste

INSTRUCTIONS

• Put the split peas and 3½ cups (840 ml) of the water in a large pot over high heat. Bring the split peas to a boil, then reduce the heat to medium and simmer, uncovered, for 30 to 40 minutes, until the split peas are tender and most of the water is absorbed. Scoop the cooked split peas from the pot into a small bowl.

• In the same large pot over medium heat, combine oil, onions, and additional 1 to 2 tablespoons (15 to 30 ml) water. Cook the onions for 5 minutes, then add the garlic and cook 2 additional minutes, stirring frequently.

• Add the split peas, vegetable stock, salt, and pepper and bring the mixture to a boil over high heat. Reduce the heat to medium, add the green tea bags, stir, and simmer, uncovered, for 5 minutes.

• Add the green peas and mint, and adjust the temperature as needed to keep the soup at a gentle simmer for 10 to 15 minutes.

• Remove the pot from the heat, remove and discard the green tea bags, and let the soup cool for 10 minutes.

• Puree the soup using a blender or immersion blender. Season the soup with additional salt, pepper, and/or mint to taste. Add the milk (if using) to make a creamy soup.

• Serve the soup garnished with an additional mint leaf.

Baked Eggs in Avocado

INGREDIENTS

• 1 large avocado

• Salt and black pepper to taste

• Curry powder to taste (optional)

• 2 large eggs

• 1 tablespoon (3 g) fresh cilantro finely chopped

• Olive oil to taste

INSTRUCTIONS

• Preheat the oven to 425°F (220°C).

• Slice the avocado in half and remove the pit. Slice a small section from the back of each half to make a flat surface in the skin, then place both halves, flesh-side up, on a small rimmed baking sheet lined with foil. Using a spoon, carefully scoop out some of the flesh to make a little more space for the eggs but don't go all the way to the skin. Place the scooped-out avocado flesh in a medium bowl and set aside.

• Sprinkle the salt and pepper and curry powder (if using) on both avocado halves. Carefully break an egg into each half, being sure not to break the yolks. Sprinkle some additional salt and pepper and curry powder (if using) on the eggs if desired.

• Bake the avocado halves for 15 minutes for a poached egg (with a runny yolk), or 18 to 20 minutes if you prefer your eggs more solid.

• While the eggs are baking, add salt, the cilantro, and olive oil to the reserved avocado. Mash lightly to make a topping for the eggs.

• Once the eggs are done, remove them from the oven and let them sit 1 minute. Place each avocado half in a bowl. Scrape up any crispy eggs that remain on the baking sheet and add them to each bowl for an extra crunch. Top the eggs with the avocado-herb mixture and eat with a spoon.

NOTES

If you've ever cut open an avocado only to realize it was too hard and not ripe yet, this is a great way to salvage it. After being baked, the avocado will end up perfectly soft, no matter how it starts out.

Don't be tempted to skip lining the baking sheet with foil; this recipe can create a very stubborn baked-on mess that takes a lot of elbow grease to clean. Trust me on this one.

Base Chicken Stock (lower your iron Hemochromatosis Cookbook)

Ingredients

• 6 green tea bags

• fatty boneless white and dark chicken or turkey meat

• 12 c water, preferably filtered

• 1 t salt

• 1 medium whole onion

• 1 large clove garlic

• 4 T fresh chopped parsley

Directions

• Simmer meat in water. Add salt, onion, garlic, parsley. Cover and simmer for at least 2-1/2 hrs. Remove meat, add tea bags to steep for 15 minutes. Remove tea bags and strain, if desired. Cool and store for use in chili, soup and stews. Servings dependent upon amount of water used.

Turkey Chili (low iron from Hemochromatosis cookbook)

Ingredients

• 1 T olive oil

• 1/2 c finely chopped onions

• 1 lb fresh ground turkey

• 1 15-1/4-oz can diced tomatoes

• 1 6-oz can tomato paste

• 2-1/4 c hot coffee

• 1 c ketchup

• 1 t salt

• 1/2 t red pepper

• 1 15-1/4 oz can dark red kidney beans

Directions

• In saucepan heat the oil and saute onion. Add meat and cook till done. Add tomatoes and simmer for 15 minutes. Add tomato paste, hot coffee, ketchup, seasonings to taste. Simmer for 30 mins. Rinse and drain beans, add to chili and heat thoroughly.

• Serve topped with sour cream, cilantro, etc.

Avocado Blueberry and Hemp Seed Smoothie (1 16-oz serving)

Ingredients

• 1 fresh medium-sized bananas (0.31mg iron)

• 1 cup baby spinach or 1 cup mixed baby kale/baby spinach (about 0.68mg iron)

• 1.5 cup frozen blueberries (0.6mg iron)

• ½ fresh, ripe avocado (0.4 mg iron)

• 1 tbsp hemp seeds – blend it into the smoothie or use as a topping (0.79mg iron)

• 1/2 -3/4 cup water (depending on how thick you'd like this to be)

TOTAL IRON CONTENT: 2.78mg (15.4% of recommended daily intake for a non-pregnant woman)

These simple smothered potatoes soak up the flavors of onion, broth and thyme as they cook in a cast-iron skillet. Be sure your cast-iron pan is well seasoned to prevent the potatoes from sticking to the pan once the liquid is absorbed.

Ingredients

• 1 tablespoon extra-virgin olive oil

• 1 cup halved and sliced onion

• 2 cloves garlic, grated

• ½ cup low-sodium chicken or vegetable broth

• ¾ teaspoon dried thyme

• ¾ teaspoon salt

• ¼ teaspoon ground pepper

• 1 ½ pounds Yukon Gold potatoes, scrubbed and sliced

• Snipped chives for garnish

Directions

• Heat oil in a large cast-iron or nonstick skillet over medium heat. Add onion and cook, stirring, until softened and beginning to brown, about 3 minutes. Add garlic and cook, stirring, until fragrant, about 30 seconds. Add broth, thyme, salt and pepper; bring to a simmer. Add potatoes in an even layer and return to a simmer; cover and cook, stirring every 5 minutes and reducing heat to maintain a gentle simmer, until the potatoes are tender and the liquid is absorbed, 15 to 20 minutes. Garnish with chives, if desired.

Nutrition Facts

Serving Size: 1 cup

Per Serving: 108 calories; protein 2g; carbohydrates 21g; dietary fiber 3g; sugars 2g; fat 2g; mono fat 2g; vitamin a iu 6IU; vitamin c 25mg; vitamin e iu 1IU; folate 4mg; vitamin k 2mg; sodium 298mg;

calcium 9mg; iron 1mg; magnesium 3mg; phosphorus 8mg; potassium 34mg.

Ingredients

• 4 tablespoons peanut oil or canola oil, divided

• 1 pound mixed mushrooms, sliced

• 1 medium red bell pepper, diced

• 1 bunch scallions, trimmed and cut into 2-inch pieces

• 1 tablespoon grated fresh ginger

• 1 large clove garlic, grated

• 1 (8 ounce) container baked tofu or smoked tofu, diced

• 3 tablespoons oyster sauce or vegetarian oyster sauce (see Tip)

Directions

• Heat 2 tablespoons oil in a large flat-bottom wok or cast-iron skillet over high heat. Add mushrooms and bell pepper; cook, stirring occasionally, until soft, about 4 minutes. Stir in scallions, ginger and garlic; cook for 30 seconds more. Transfer the vegetables to a bowl.

• Add the remaining 2 tablespoons oil and tofu to the pan. Cook, turning once, until browned, 3 to 4 minutes. Stir in the vegetables and oyster sauce. Cook, stirring, until hot, about 1 minute.

Tips

Tip: Sweet, salty oyster sauce is made from, well, oysters, along with salt, sugar and sometimes soy sauce. Substitute vegetarian oyster or stir-fry sauce, if desired, which uses mushrooms instead of oysters.

Balsamic-Parmesan Sautéed Spinach

Ingredients

• 2 tablespoons extra-virgin olive oil

• 3 cloves garlic, minced

• 1 pound fresh spinach

• ¼ teaspoon salt

- ¼ teaspoon ground pepper

- 2 tablespoons grated Parmesan cheese

- 4 teaspoons good-quality balsamic vinegar or balsamic glaze

Directions

- Heat oil in a large pot over medium heat. Add garlic and cook, stirring, until fragrant, 30 seconds to 1 minute. Add spinach, salt and pepper; toss to coat. Cook, stirring, until just wilted, 3 to 5 minutes. Remove from heat and stir in Parmesan. Drizzle with vinegar (or glaze) and serve immediately.

Nutrition Facts

Serving Size: 1/2 cup

Per Serving: 84 calories; protein 3.3g; carbohydrates 5g; dietary fiber 2.1g; sugars 1g; fat 6.3g; saturated fat 1.1g; cholesterol 1.7mg; vitamin a iu 8526.9IU; vitamin c 26mg; folate 176.2mcg; calcium 111.9mg; iron 2.6mg; magnesium 73.5mg; potassium 523.4mg; sodium 225.4mg; thiamin 0.1mg.

Ingredients

• 12 ounces boneless beef top sirloin steak, cut 1 inch thick and trimmed

• 2 teaspoons salt-free steak grilling seasoning, such as Mrs. Dash®

• 2 cloves garlic, minced

• ½ teaspoon salt, divided

• 2 teaspoons canola oil

• 6 ounces broccolini, trimmed

• 2 cups frozen peas

• 1 teaspoon chopped fresh thyme

• 3 cups sliced fresh mushrooms

• 1 cup unsalted beef broth

• 1 tablespoon whole-grain mustard

• 2 teaspoons cornstarch

Directions

• Preheat oven to 350°F. Sprinkle steak with steak seasoning, garlic and 1/4 teaspoon salt. Heat oil in a 12-inch cast-iron skillet over medium-high heat. Add the steak and broccolini. Cook for 4 minutes, turning the broccolini once (do not turn the steak). Place peas around the steak; sprinkle with thyme. Transfer the skillet to oven and bake until the steak is medium-rare (145°F), about 8 minutes. Transfer the steak and vegetables to a plate (leave the drippings in the pan); cover and keep warm.

• Add mushrooms to the drippings in the pan. Cook over medium-high heat for 3 minutes, stirring occasionally. Whisk broth, mustard, cornstarch and the remaining ¼ teaspoon salt in a small bowl or measuring cup; add to the pan with the mushrooms. Cook, stirring, until thick and bubbly, about 1 to 2 minutes. Cook, stirring, for 1 minute more. Serve the steak and vegetables with the sauce.

Nutrition Facts

Serving Size: 2 1/2 ounces meat and 1/3 cup sauce

Per Serving: 231 calories; protein 26g; carbohydrates 18g; dietary fiber 4g; sugars 5g; fat 7g; saturated fat 2g; cholesterol 51mg; vitamin a iu 2139IU; vitamin c 53mg; folate 56mcg; calcium 71mg; iron 3mg; magnesium 43mg; potassium 719mg; sodium 520mg.

Eggplant & Chickpea Baked Pasta

Ingredients

• 8 ounces whole-wheat fusilli

• ½ cup coarse dry whole-wheat breadcrumbs (see Note)

• 1 tablespoon extra-virgin olive oil

• 3 cups Eggplant & Chickpea Stew (see associated recipe)

• 1 cup crumbled feta cheese

• ½ cup chopped fresh mint or basil, divided

• 2 tablespoons lemon juice

Directions

• Preheat oven to 350 degrees F. Coat an 8-inch-square (or similar 2-quart) baking dish with cooking spray.

• Bring a large pot of water to a boil. Cook pasta according to package directions. Drain and rinse.

• Combine breadcrumbs and oil in a small bowl. Toss the pasta with stew, feta, 1/4 cup mint (or basil) and lemon juice in a large bowl. Spread the mixture in the prepared baking dish. Top with the breadcrumb mixture.

• Bake until the topping is golden and crispy, about 30 minutes. Sprinkle with the remaining 1/4 cup mint (or basil).

Sheet-Pan Steak & Potatoes

Ingredients

• 1 pound potatoes, cut into 1/2-inch wedges

• 2 tablespoons extra-virgin olive oil, divided

• ¾ teaspoon salt, divided

• ¾ teaspoon ground pepper, divided

• 4 cups chopped asparagus

• 1 ¼ pounds skirt steak, trimmed

• ½ teaspoon garlic powder

• ½ teaspoon dried rosemary

• 3 tablespoons crumbled blue cheese

Directions

• Preheat oven to 425 degrees F.

• Toss potatoes with 1 tablespoon oil and 1/4 teaspoon each salt and pepper in a large bowl. Spread evenly on a rimmed baking sheet. Roast for 15 minutes.

• Toss asparagus with the remaining 1 tablespoon oil and 1/4 teaspoon each salt and pepper in the bowl. Stir into the potatoes on the baking sheet.

• Sprinkle steak with garlic powder, rosemary and the remaining 1/4 teaspoon each salt and pepper. Place on top of the vegetables. Roast until the steak is cooked and the vegetables are tender, 10 to 15 minutes more.

• Transfer the steak to a serving platter. Stir blue cheese into the vegetables and serve with the steak.

Nutrition Facts

Serving Size: 1 cup vegetables & 4 oz. steak

Per Serving: 415 calories; protein 35.1g; carbohydrates 21.5g; dietary fiber 3.5g; sugars 2.4g; fat 20.8g; saturated fat 6.7g; cholesterol 96.9mg; vitamin a iu 723.7IU; vitamin c 14.9mg; folate 131.5mcg; calcium 75.7mg; iron 4.7mg; magnesium 66.8mg; potassium 1214.7mg; sodium 633.5mg.

Tofu, Mushroom & Bok Choy Soba Noodle Bowls

Ingredients

• 3 tablespoons canola oil, divided

• 2 teaspoons toasted sesame oil

• 1 teaspoon grated fresh ginger

- 2 cloves garlic, grated

- 4 scallions, sliced, greens and whites separated, divided

- 1 serrano pepper, thinly sliced

- 4 cups low-sodium no-chicken broth (see Tip)

- 2 tablespoons reduced-sodium tamari or soy sauce (see Tip)

- 2 heads baby bok choy, thinly sliced

- 5 ounces sliced shiitake mushroom caps

- ¼ teaspoon salt

- 8 ounces buckwheat soba or udon noodles

- 1 (14 ounce) package extra-firm tofu, drained and cut into bite-size cubes

- Fresh cilantro for garnish

Directions

- Bring a medium saucepan of water to a boil.

• Heat 1 tablespoon canola oil in a large saucepan over medium heat. Add sesame oil, ginger, garlic, scallion whites and serrano and cook until fragrant, about 1 minute. Add broth and tamari (or soy sauce) and bring to a boil. Cover and simmer while you prepare vegetables and noodles.

• Heat the remaining 2 tablespoons canola oil in a large skillet or flat-bottom wok over high heat. Add bok choy and shiitakes and cook, stirring occasionally, until well browned, about 8 minutes. Sprinkle with salt. Remove from heat.

• Cook noodles in the boiling water according to package directions. Drain and divide among 4 serving bowls. Top with the vegetables and tofu and ladle on the hot broth. Top with scallion greens and garnish with cilantro, if desired.

Tips

Slightly less sweet than the average vegetable broth, no-chicken broth has a more savory flavor thanks to the addition of spices meant to mimic chicken broth. Opt for the low-sodium version to save 380 mg per serving.

People with celiac disease or gluten sensitivity should use soy sauces that are labeled "gluten-free," as soy sauce may contain wheat or other gluten-containing ingredients.

Nutrition Facts

Serving Size: 2 cups

Per Serving: 459 calories; fat 19g; sodium 706mg; carbohydrates 54g; dietary fiber 7g; protein 20g; sugars 6g; niacin equivalents 2mg; saturated fat 2g; vitamin a iu 4301IU; potassium 576mg.

Kale & Quinoa Salad with Lemon Dressing

Ingredients

• 1 bunch lacinato kale, stemmed and chopped

• 6 tablespoons extra-virgin olive oil

• 3 tablespoons lemon juice

• 2 tablespoons chopped shallot

• 1 teaspoon honey

• ½ teaspoon salt

• ¼ teaspoon ground pepper

• 2 cups grape or cherry tomatoes, halved

• 2 cups cooked quinoa

• 1 English cucumber, thinly sliced

• 1 medium red bell pepper, sliced

• 1 medium yellow bell pepper, sliced

• 1 (15 ounce) can unsalted chickpeas, rinsed

• ¾ cup feta cheese, crumbled

• ½ cup sliced almonds, toasted

Directions

• Place kale in a large serving bowl. Whisk together oil, lemon juice, shallot, honey, salt and pepper in a small bowl. Pour 2 to 3 tablespoons of the dressing over the kale; lightly massage until slightly wilted, 1 to 2 minutes.

• Top the kale with tomatoes, quinoa, cucumber, peppers, chickpeas, feta and almonds. Drizzle with the remaining dressing and toss before serving.

To make ahead

Refrigerate in an airtight container for up to 3 days.

Nutrition Facts

Serving Size: 1 3/4 cups

Per Serving: 400 calories; fat 23g; cholesterol 5mg; sodium 406mg; carbohydrates 37g; dietary fiber 8g; protein 14g; sugars 6g; niacin equivalents 1mg; saturated fat 4g; vitamin a iu 3984IU; potassium 594mg.

Lentil & Goat Cheese Toast

Ingredients

• 2 tablespoons goat cheese

• 2 slices olive sourdough bread, toasted

• .666 cup rinsed canned French green lentils

• 2 tablespoons chopped walnuts, toasted

Directions

• Spread 1 tablespoon goat cheese on each slice of toast. Top each with 1/3 cup lentils and 1 tablespoon walnuts.

Nutrition Facts

Serving Size: 1 toast

Per Serving: 282 calories; fat 11g; cholesterol 42mg; sodium 352mg; carbohydrates 35g; dietary fiber 6g; protein 11g; sugars 1g; niacin equivalents 1mg; saturated fat 2g; vitamin a iu 2IU; potassium 270mg.

Vegetarian Potato-Kale Soup

Ingredients

• 1 tablespoon extra-virgin olive oil

• 1 small sweet onion, halved and thinly sliced

• 3 cloves garlic, finely chopped

• 4 cups low-sodium vegetable broth

• 2 cups water

• 1 pound baby red potatoes, halved lengthwise

• 2 medium parsnips, peeled and sliced 1/4-inch thick

• 1 teaspoon chopped fresh rosemary, plus more for garnish

• ¼ teaspoon salt

• 1 small bunch lacinato kale, stemmed and chopped

• ½ cup grated Parmesan cheese, plus more for garnish

• ¼ cup heavy cream

• 1 tablespoon lemon juice

Directions

• Heat oil in a Dutch oven or large heavy pot over medium-high heat. Add onion; cook, stirring occasionally, under tender, about 5 minutes. Add garlic; cook, stirring constantly, until fragrant, about 30 seconds. Stir in broth, water, potatoes, parsnips, rosemary and salt; bring to a boil. Reduce heat to medium-low; cover and cook, stirring occasionally, until the vegetables are tender, about 15 minutes. Using the back of a spoon, gently mash the vegetables to slightly thicken the soup.

• Stir in kale, Parmesan and cream; cook over medium-low heat, stirring occasionally, until the kale is wilted, about 10 minutes more. Stir in lemon juice just before serving. Garnish with additional rosemary and Parmesan, if desired.

Nutrition Facts

Serving Size: 2 cups

Per Serving: 273 calories; fat 12g; cholesterol 23mg; sodium 444mg; carbohydrates 38g; dietary fiber 7g; protein 7g; sugars 7g;

niacin equivalents 2mg; saturated fat 5g; vitamin a iu 4103IU; potassium 913mg.

Pan-Seared Steak with Crispy Herbs & Escarole

Ingredients

• 1 pound sirloin steak, about 1/2 inch thick

• ½ teaspoon salt, divided

• ½ teaspoon ground pepper, divided

• 2 tablespoons grapeseed oil or canola oil

• 4 cloves garlic, crushed

• 5 sprigs fresh thyme

• 3 sprigs fresh sage

• 1 sprig fresh rosemary

• 16 cups chopped escarole (about 1 pound)

Directions

• Sprinkle steak with 1/4 teaspoon each salt and pepper. Heat a large cast-iron skillet over medium-high heat. Add the steak and cook until charred on one side, about 3 minutes. Turn the steak over and add oil, garlic, thyme, sage and rosemary. Cook, stirring the herbs occasionally, until an instant-read thermometer inserted in the thickest part of the steak reaches 125 degrees F for medium-rare, 3 to 4 minutes. Transfer the steak to a plate and top with the garlic and herbs. Tent with foil.

• Add escarole and the remaining 1/4 teaspoon each salt and pepper to the pan. Cook, stirring often, until the escarole starts to wilt, about 2 minutes. Thinly slice the steak and serve with the escarole and crispy herbs.

Nutrition Facts

Serving Size: 3 oz. meat, 1/2 cup escarole and 1/2 Tbsp. herbs

Per Serving: 244 calories; protein 25.5g; carbohydrates 10g; dietary fiber 8.2g; sugars 0.7g; fat 11.8g; saturated fat 2.5g; cholesterol 59.2mg; vitamin a iu 5606.1IU; vitamin c 18.6mg; folate 373.3mcg;

calcium 160.1mg; iron 3.7mg; magnesium 60.3mg; potassium 1110.5mg; sodium 393.6mg.

Ingredients

• 2 tablespoons lemon juice

• 1 tablespoon nonpareil capers, rinsed and chopped

• 1 tablespoon finely chopped shallot

• ¼ teaspoon salt

• ¼ teaspoon ground pepper

• 1 (15 ounce) can no-salt-added chickpeas, rinsed

• 1 (6.7 ounce) jar oil-packed tuna, drained

• 1 cup halved cherry tomatoes

• 1 cup thinly sliced English cucumber

• ½ cup crumbled feta cheese

• 2 tablespoons chopped fresh dill

• 3 tablespoons extra-virgin olive oil

• 3 cups baby spinach

Directions

• Stir lemon juice, capers, shallot, salt and pepper together in a large bowl. Let stand for 5 minutes.

• Meanwhile, toss chickpeas, tuna, tomatoes, cucumber, feta and dill together in a large bowl.

• Whisk oil into the lemon juice mixture until fully incorporated. Spoon about 5 tablespoons of the dressing into the chickpea mixture; toss to coat.

• Add spinach to the remaining dressing in the large bowl; toss to coat. Divide the spinach evenly among 4 plates; top each plate with 1 1/4 cups chickpea mixture. Serve immediately.

To make ahead

• Prepare through Step 3 and refrigerate in an airtight container for up to 1 day.

Nutrition Facts

Serving Size: 3/4 cup spinach & 1 1/4 cups chickpea mixture

Per Serving: 357 calories; fat 19g; cholesterol 30mg; sodium 555mg; carbohydrates 23g; dietary fiber 6g; protein 21g; sugars 3g; niacin equivalents 6mg; saturated fat 5g; vitamin a iu 1869IU; potassium 505mg.

Gochujang Steak with Roasted Potatoes & Broccolini

Ingredients

• 1 ½ pounds fingerling potatoes, halved or quartered lengthwise, depending on size

• 3 tablespoons extra-virgin olive oil, divided

• ¼ teaspoon salt, divided

• ¼ teaspoon ground pepper, divided

• 1 medium apple, coarsely chopped

• ½ medium onion, coarsely chopped

• 2 scallions, chopped, whites and greens separated

• 2 cloves garlic, coarsely chopped

• 3 tablespoons brown sugar

• 2 tablespoons gochujang

• 2 tablespoons low-sodium soy sauce

• 1 tablespoon rice vinegar

• 1 pound steak tips

• 1 pound broccolini, trimmed

Directions

• Position racks in upper and lower thirds of oven. Place a large rimmed baking sheet on the lower rack. Preheat oven to 425°F. Line another baking sheet with foil.

• Toss potatoes with 2 tablespoons oil and 1/8 teaspoon each salt and pepper in a medium bowl. Carefully transfer to the hot baking sheet.

Roast on the lower rack, flipping once, until the potatoes are browned and tender, about 35 minutes.

• Meanwhile, combine apple, onion, scallion whites, garlic, brown sugar, gochujang, soy sauce and vinegar in a blender. Puree until smooth. Reserve 1/2 cup for serving and pour the rest into the bowl; add steak tips and toss to coat. Marinate at room temperature for 10 minutes.

• Combine broccolini, the remaining 1 tablespoon oil and 1/8 teaspoon each salt and pepper in a medium bowl; toss to coat.

• Arrange the broccolini on one side of the foil-lined baking sheet and the steak on the other side. Roast on the upper rack until the broccolini is tender and an instant-read thermometer inserted in the thickest part of the steak registers 125°F for medium-rare, 10 to 14 minutes. Turn the broiler to high and broil until the broccolini and steak start to brown, 1 to 2 minutes.

• Serve the steak with the broccolini, potatoes and reserved sauce. Garnish with scallion greens.

Nutrition Facts

Serving Size: 3 oz. steak, 1 cup each potatoes and broccolini & 2 Tbsp. sauce

White Bean Soup with Pasta

Ingredients

• 1 tablespoon extra-virgin olive oil

• 1 ½ cups frozen mirepoix (diced onion, celery and carrot)

• 2 cloves garlic, minced

• 1 teaspoon Italian seasoning

• 1 teaspoon salt

• ¼ teaspoon crushed red pepper

• ¼ teaspoon ground pepper

• 1 (28 ounce) can no-salt-added diced tomatoes

• 2 cups low-sodium no-chicken broth or chicken broth

• 1 (15-ounce) can low-sodium cannellini beans, rinsed

• 8 ounces small whole-wheat pasta, such as elbows

• 1 ½ cups frozen cut-leaf spinach

• 4 tablespoons grated Parmesan cheese

Directions

• Put a large saucepan of water on to boil.

• Heat oil in a large pot over medium-high heat. Add mirepoix and cook, stirring, until softened, about 3 minutes. Add garlic, Italian seasoning, salt, crushed red pepper and ground pepper and cook, stirring, until fragrant, about 1 minute. Add tomatoes and their juices, broth and beans and bring to a boil. Reduce heat to maintain a lively simmer. Cover and cook, stirring occasionally, until the tomatoes begin to break down, about 10 minutes.

• Meanwhile, cook pasta in the boiling water for 1 minute less than the package directions. Drain.

• Stir spinach into the soup. Stir in the pasta just before serving. Serve topped with Parmesan.

To make ahead

Refrigerate soup and pasta separately for up to 3 days.

Nutrition Facts

Serving Size: 1 1/3 cups

Per Serving: 277 calories; fat 5g; cholesterol 3mg; sodium 576mg; carbohydrates 49g; dietary fiber 9g; protein 12g; sugars 7g; niacin equivalents 3mg; saturated fat 1g; vitamin a iu 2217IU; potassium 329mg.

Vegan Lentil Stew

Ingredients

• 2 tablespoons extra-virgin olive oil, divided

• 1 large sweet potato (12 ounces), unpeeled and cut into 1/2-inch pieces

• 2 medium leeks, thinly sliced into half-moons

• 2 large carrots, roughly chopped

• 3 cloves garlic, minced

• 2 tablespoons tomato paste

• 1 ½ teaspoons ground cumin

• 1 ¼ teaspoons white miso

• 6 cups water

• 1 ½ cups green or brown lentils

• ½ teaspoon salt

• 4 cups chopped hearty greens, such as kale or Swiss chard

Directions

• Heat 1 tablespoon oil in a large Dutch oven over medium-high heat. Add sweet potato; cook, stirring occasionally, until lightly browned and beginning to soften, 6 to 8 minutes. Add leeks and carrots; cook, stirring occasionally, until softened, 3 to 4 minutes. Stir in garlic, tomato paste, cumin, miso and the remaining 1 tablespoon oil; cook, stirring constantly, until fragrant and the tomato paste has darkened, about 1 minute.

• Add water, lentils and salt; bring to a boil over high heat. Reduce heat to medium-low; cover and cook until the lentils are almost tender, 25 minutes. Stir in greens; cover and cook until the greens are wilted, about 10 minutes.

To make ahead

Refrigerate in an airtight container for up to 1 week or freeze for up to 3 months.

Nutrition Facts

Serving Size: 2 cups

Per Serving: 451 calories; fat 8g; sodium 475mg; carbohydrates 77g; dietary fiber 13g; protein 22g; sugars 9g; niacin equivalents 3mg; saturated fat 1g; vitamin a iu 24966IU; potassium 964mg.

Scallion-Ginger Beef & Broccoli

Ingredients

• ⅓ cup reduced-sodium tamari or soy sauce

- ¼ cup low-sodium chicken broth

- 2 tablespoons brown sugar

- 2 tablespoons cornstarch, divided

- 1 pound sirloin steak, thinly sliced

- 3 tablespoons peanut or canola oil, divided

- 6 cups broccoli florets

- ½ cup sliced scallions, plus more for garnish

- 1 tablespoon finely grated ginger

- 1 teaspoon finely grated garlic

- 2 cups cooked brown rice

- Crushed red pepper for garnish

Directions

- Whisk tamari (or soy sauce), broth, brown sugar and 1 tablespoon cornstarch in a small bowl. Toss steak with the remaining 1 tablespoon cornstarch.

• Heat 2 tablespoons oil in a large flat-bottom wok or cast-iron skillet over medium-high heat. Add the steak and cook, stirring once, until browned, about 4 minutes. Transfer to a clean plate. Add the remaining 1 tablespoon oil and broccoli; cook, stirring occasionally, until slightly tender, about 2 minutes. Stir in scallions, ginger and garlic; cook, stirring, until fragrant, about 30 seconds. Whisk the tamari mixture and add it, along with the beef, back to the pan; cook until the sauce thickens, about 1 minute. Serve over brown rice and garnish with crushed red pepper, if desired.

Nutrition Facts

Serving Size: 1 cup beef & broccoli & 1/2 cup rice

Per Serving: 441 calories; protein 30g; carbohydrates 43.2g; dietary fiber 4.5g; sugars 8.9g; fat 16g; saturated fat 3.7g; cholesterol 59.2mg; vitamin a iu 3319.7IU; vitamin c 101.9mg; folate 101.2mcg; calcium 85.3mg; iron 4.7mg; magnesium 89mg; potassium 780.7mg; sodium 741mg; thiamin 0.3mg.

Ingredients

- ½ cup plain low-fat Greek yogurt

- ¼ cup crumbled feta cheese

- 1 tablespoon lemon juice

- ¼ teaspoon honey

- 1 tablespoon chopped fresh dill, divided, plus more for garnish

- 1 tablespoon thinly sliced chives, divided, plus more for garnish

- 2 teaspoons finely chopped garlic, divided

- 1 (15 ounce) can unsalted chickpeas, rinsed

- ⅓ cup chickpea flour

- 1 tablespoon tahini

- ½ teaspoon ground cumin

- ½ teaspoon ground coriander

• 1 large egg, lightly beaten

• ½ teaspoon salt

• 3 tablespoons canola oil, divided

Directions

• Combine yogurt, feta, lemon juice, honey and 1 teaspoon each dill, chives and garlic in a medium bowl; stir until blended. Refrigerate until ready to serve.

• Place chickpeas in a large bowl and mash with the back of a fork or a potato masher until almost smooth but some chunks remain. Add chickpea flour, tahini, cumin, coriander, egg, salt and the remaining 2 teaspoons each dill and chives and 1 teaspoon garlic; stir until combined.

• Heat 1 1/2 tablespoons oil in a large nonstick skillet over medium-high heat. Working with half of the chickpea mixture at a time, scoop even tablespoonfuls into the hot skillet; use the back of a spoon dipped in water to press down slightly to flatten into about 2-inch-diameter cakes. Cook, turning once, until golden brown on both sides, about 1 to 2 minutes per side. Transfer to a paper-towel-lined plate. Repeat with the remaining oil and chickpea mixture. Serve with the yogurt-feta dip; garnish with dill and chives, if desired.

Nutrition Facts

Serving Size: 3 fritters & 2 Tbsp. dip

Per Serving: 223 calories; fat 12g; cholesterol 39mg; sodium 289mg; carbohydrates 19g; dietary fiber 4g; protein 10g; sugars 3g; niacin equivalents 1mg; saturated fat 2g; vitamin a iu 161IU; potassium 191mg.

Mussels with White Beans & Tomatoes

Ingredients

• 2 tablespoons extra-virgin olive oil

• 4 cups grape tomatoes, halved

• 1 medium shallot, sliced

• 3 cloves garlic, thinly sliced

• 1 teaspoon chopped fresh thyme, plus more for garnish

• ¼ teaspoon crushed red pepper

• 1 (15 ounce) can no-salt-added white beans, rinsed

• 2 pounds mussels, scrubbed and debearded if necessary (see Tip)

• ½ cup dry white wine

• Lemon wedges for serving

Directions

• Heat oil in a large pot over medium-high heat. Add tomatoes and shallot; cook, stirring occasionally, until the tomatoes start to release their liquid, 1 to 2 minutes. Stir in garlic, thyme and crushed red pepper; cook until fragrant, about 1 minute. Add beans and stir to combine. Place mussels on top and pour in wine. Cover and cook until the mussels open (discard any unopened mussels), 5 to 6 minutes. Serve with lemon wedges and garnish with more thyme, if desired.

Tips

Tip: To clean mussels, rinse very well under cold running water and use a stiff brush to remove any barnacles or grit from the shell. Discard any mussels with broken shells or any shells that remain open after you tap them lightly. Pull off any fibrous "beard" that might be pinched between the shells; the "beards" of most cultivated mussels are already removed.

Nutrition Facts

Serving Size: 10 mussels & 1 cup broth

Per Serving: 395 calories; protein 33.8g; carbohydrates 37.6g; dietary fiber 5.9g; sugars 2.5g; fat 12.9g; saturated fat 2g; cholesterol 63.5mg; vitamin a iu 1478.9IU; vitamin c 37.7mg; folate 97.5mcg; calcium 98.5mg; iron 10.5mg; magnesium 127.2mg; potassium 963.3mg; sodium 711.1mg.

Exchanges: 4 lean protein, 3 vegetable, 1 1/2 fat, 1 starch

Ravioli & Vegetable Soup

Ingredients

• 1 tablespoon extra-virgin olive oil

• 2 cups frozen bell pepper and onion mix, thawed and diced

• 2 cloves garlic, minced

• 1/4 teaspoon crushed red pepper, or to taste (optional)

• 1 28-ounce can crushed tomatoes, preferably fire-roasted

• 1 15-ounce can vegetable broth or reduced-sodium chicken broth

• 1 ½ cups hot water

• 1 teaspoon dried basil or marjoram

• 1 6- to 9-ounce package fresh or frozen cheese (or meat) ravioli, preferably whole-wheat

• 2 cups diced zucchini, (about 2 medium)

• Freshly ground pepper to taste

Directions

• Heat oil in a large saucepan or Dutch oven over medium heat. Add pepper-onion mix, garlic and crushed red pepper (if using) and cook, stirring, for 1 minute. Add tomatoes, broth, water and basil (or marjoram); bring to a rolling boil over high heat. Add ravioli and cook for 3 minutes less than the package directions. Add zucchini; return to a boil. Cook until the zucchini is crisp-tender, about 3 minutes. Season with pepper.

Tips

Make Ahead Tip: Cover and refrigerate for up to 3 days. Thin with broth before reheating, if desired.

Nutrition Facts

Serving Size: about 2 cups

Per Serving: 261 calories; protein 10.6g; carbohydrates 32.6g; dietary fiber 7g; sugars 11.8g; fat 8.3g; saturated fat 3g; cholesterol 28.4mg; vitamin a iu 2278.7IU; vitamin c 23.9mg; folate 16mcg; calcium 97.4mg; iron 5mg; magnesium 15mg; potassium 731.9mg; sodium 354.4mg.

Exchanges: 1 starch, 2 vegetable, 1 fat

Ingredients

• ½ cup sliced oil-packed sun-dried tomatoes plus 2 tablespoons oil from the jar, divided

• 1 (16 ounce) package shelf-stable gnocchi

• 1 (15 ounce) can low-sodium cannellini beans, rinsed

• 1 (5 ounce) package baby spinach

• 1 large shallot, minced

• ⅓ cup low-sodium no-chicken broth or chicken broth

• ⅓ cup heavy cream

• 1 tablespoon lemon juice

• ¼ teaspoon salt

• ¼ teaspoon ground pepper

• 3 tablespoons fresh basil leaves

Directions

• Heat 1 tablespoon oil in a large nonstick skillet over medium-high heat. Add gnocchi and cook, stirring often, until plumped and starting to brown, about 5 minutes. Add beans and spinach and cook until the spinach is wilted, about 1 minute. Transfer to a plate.

• Add the remaining 1 tablespoon oil to the pan and heat over medium heat. Add sun-dried tomatoes and shallot; cook, stirring, for 1 minute. Increase heat to high and add broth. Cook until the liquid has mostly evaporated, about 2 minutes.

• Reduce heat to medium and stir in cream, lemon juice, salt and pepper. Return the gnocchi mixture to the pan and stir to coat with the sauce. Serve topped with basil.